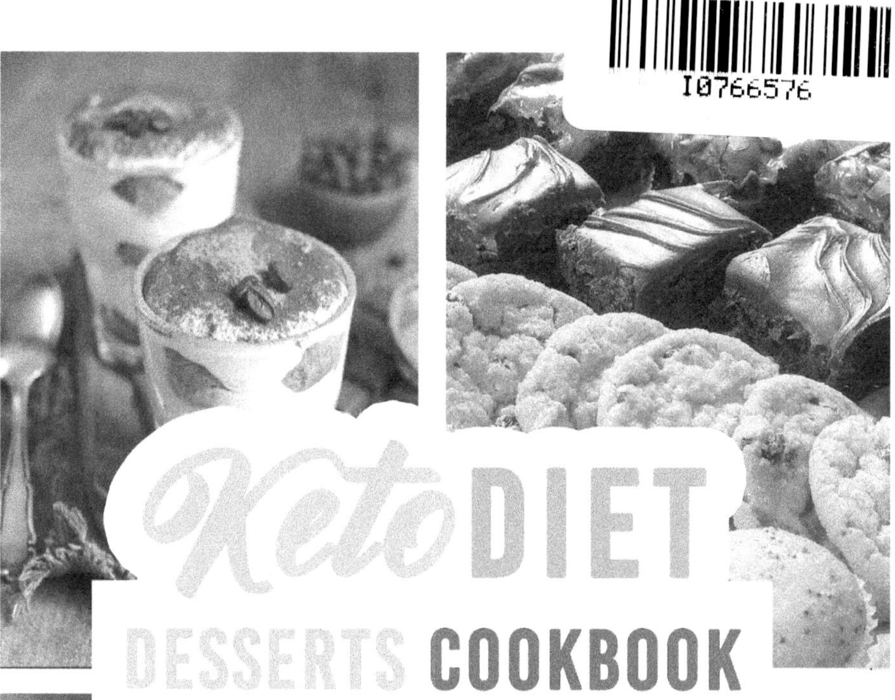

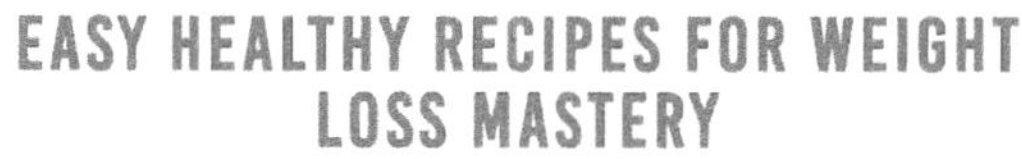

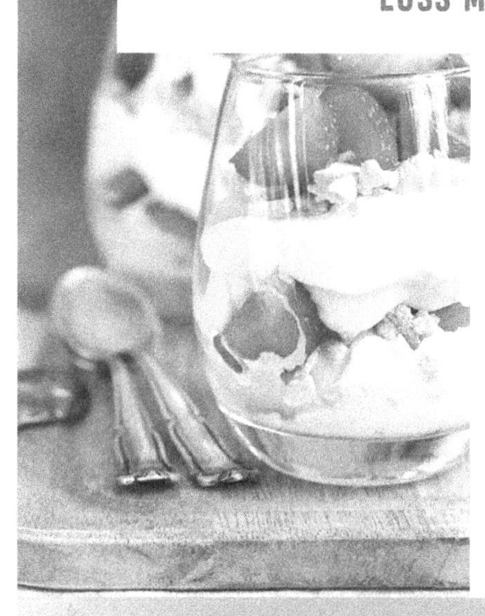

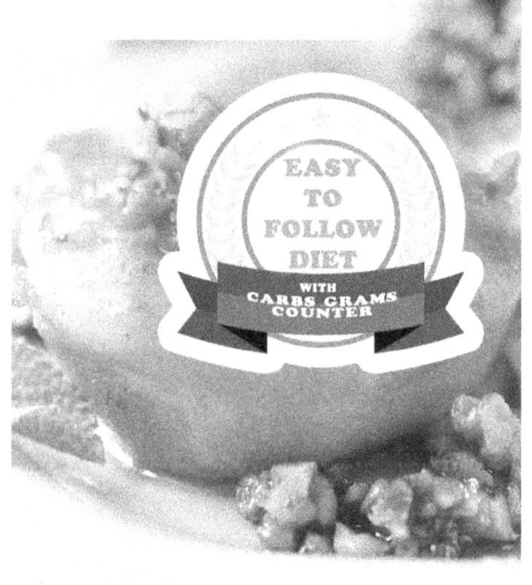

JASON STEPHENS

This content is provided with the only purpose of providing relevant information on a specific topic for which every reasonable effort has been made to ensure that it's both accurate and correct. Nevertheless, by purchasing this book, you consent that the Author and the Publisher are not experts or professionals about these topics, regardless of any claims they made within. So, any suggestions or recommendations made inside this book have mere entertainment value. We recommend that you always consult a professional before undertaking any of the advice or techniques discussed inside this title.

This declaration is legally binding within the United States and must be considered valid and fair by both the Committee of Publishers Association and the American Bar Association.

No part of this publication may be reproduced, distributed, or transmitted in any form or by any means, including photocopying, recording, or other electronic or mechanical methods, without the prior written permission of the Publisher, except in the case of brief quotations embodied in critical reviews and specific other noncommercial uses permitted by copyright law.

Author and Publisher cannot be considered responsible for any use of the provided content, and both can't be deemed liable for any damages or injury that may result from any misuse of the information delivered with this book.

Additionally, all the information following is intended for informational purposes only and is presented without assurance regarding its prolonged validity or interim quality. Trademarks mentioned are done without written consent and can in no way be considered an endorsement from the trademark holder.

TABLE OF CONTENT

ABOUT THE BOOK

The Keto Diet recipe for dessert cookbook features 30 low-carb, high-fat recipes designed to help make the ketogenic diet work for your individual's unique needs. The book begins with an overview of what keto diet is and the potential benefits of the diet. The cookbook walks you through the steps of setting macros and figuring out which foods items you can eat as dessert. Following that is a varied and delicious collection of recipes for lunches and dinners. The recipes are packed with handy extras that make them even easier to follow and adapt, from serving sizes to comprehensive nutrition information. With The Keto Diet Cookbook, you will find nourishing and mouthwatering ways to honor, trust, and nourish your body while enjoying your dessert.

WHAT IS KETO DIET?

The ketogenic diet, popularly called the keto diet, is a popular diet containing high amounts of fats, adequate-protein, and low carbohydrate. It is also referred to as a Low Carb-High Fat (LCHF) diet and a low carbohydrate diet. The ketogenic diet is a diet super high in fat (about 80 percent of your daily calories), super low in carbohydrates (less than 5 percent of your calories), and moderate in protein (typically 15 to 20 percent of your calories). This is a drastic departure from the generally recommended macronutrient distribution of 20 to 35 percent protein, 45 to 65 percent carbohydrates, and 10 to 35 percent fat. The most important component of the keto diet is a natural and normal process called ketosis. Normally, bodies run very well on glucose. Glucose is produced when the body breaks down carbohydrates. It's a very simple process, which is why it's the body's preferred way to produce energy.

When you cut back on carbs or just haven't eaten in a while, your body looks for other sources of energy to fill the void. Fat is typically that source. When your blood sugar drops because you're not feeding your body carbs, fat is released from your cells and flood the liver. The liver turns the fat into ketone bodies, which your body uses as its second choice for energy.

WHAT ARE THE POTENTIAL BENEFITS OF KETO DIET?

While the keto diet certainly is not easy, research shows it has some potential therapeutic benefits, in addition to its use for treating epilepsy. Here, some areas of research where a keto diet shows promise.

Keto Diet Help with Weight Loss

This is one of the keto diet's main selling points and a primary reason it's so popular: keto diet proponents say you can drop a lot of weight in a relatively short period of time. A number of studies, including one meta-analysis, have found that patients assigned to a very-low-carbohydrate diet (like the keto diet) had greater weight-loss outcomes compared with those eating low-fat.

Alzheimer's Disease

Research suggests that when patients with Alzheimer's eat a ketogenic diet, cognitive function significantly improves. It's believed that this has something to do with improving mitochondrial function by providing the brain with new fuel.

Parkinson's Disease

One of the key features of Parkinson's disease is the abnormal accumulation of a protein known as alpha-synuclein. Research has explored that a ketogenic diet stimulates the breakdown of these proteins, reducing the amount of alpha-synuclein in the brain.

Multiple Sclerosis

In a study, patients with multiple sclerosis (MS) were put on a ketogenic diet. After six months, they reported improved quality of life, as well as physical and mental health improvements. Before doctors or researchers can make a connection between keto and MS, they need bigger sample sizes and more thorough research. Still, the preliminary findings are exciting.

Type 2 Diabetes

This population has been studied heavily with the keto diet since it's technically as low-carb as you can get. While the research to date has been conducted in very small sample sizes, evidence suggests that the keto diet may help reduce A1C and improve insulin sensitivity by as much as 75 percent. A 2017 review found that a keto diet was associated with better glucose control and a reduction in medication use.

Cancer

Early experimental research suggests that the keto diet may have anti-tumor effects, likely because it reduces overall calorie intake (and circulating glucose) for tumor growth. In one 2014 review of animal research, a ketogenic diet was found to be successful at reducing tumor growth, colon cancer, gastric cancer, and brain cancer.

DEFINITION OF DESSERT

Dessert is the kind of food that concludes a meal. They consist mainly of sweet foods and most times they come as beverages. In some parts of the world, examples are Africa and china have no tradition of dessert to conclude a meal.

Desserts can mean confections such as cakes, biscuits, cookies, custards, ice creams, pies, sweet soups, and tarts, etc. Fruits are found majorly in dessert because of their natural sweetness.

30 KETO DIET RECIPES FOR DESSERTS

KETO CHOCOLATE CAKE WITH CHOCOLATE GLAZE

calories	Protein	Fats	Fiber	Carbohydrates
321	6.5g	30g	5.5g	22.4g

Prep time (start to end):40 minutes

Servings: 8

INGREDIENTS

CHOCOLATE CAKE INGREDIENTS:

- 1/2 cup coconut flour
- 5 eggs, separated
- 1/2 cup coconut oil or grass-fed ghee, melted
- 1/2 cup coconut cream
- 2 teaspoons vanilla extract, or 1 teaspoon vanilla powder
- 4 tablespoons granulated sweetener (or more to taste), such as birch xylitol, non-GMO erythritol, or MitoSweet
- 1/2 cup cacao powder
- Pinch of salt
- Additional grass-fed butter, ghee, or coconut oil for greasing

CHOCOLATE GLAZE INGREDIENTS:

- 1 cup coconut cream (from a BPA-free can of full-fat coconut milk)
- 1 tablespoon ghee or coconut oil
- 1 teaspoon vanilla extract
- 1 tablespoon cacao powder
- 1 tablespoon erythritol, xylitol, or MitoSweet, or roughly 10 drops of liquid stevia
- Pinch of salt

HOW TO MAKE

1. Preheat oven to 350 degrees. Grease an 8-inch metal cake pan with butter, ghee, or coconut oil.
2. Whisk egg whites until they develop a foamy consistency.
3. In a separate bowl, mix all remaining chocolate cake ingredients. Then slowly fold egg whites into the batter.
4. Pour batter into cake pan. Bake for 25 minutes, or until a knife inserted into the center of the cake comes out clean.
5. While keto chocolate cake cools, prepare the glaze. In a saucepan on low heat, add all glaze ingredients and whisk continuously to combine.
6. Pour chocolate glaze into a glass jar and drizzle over the cake. Serve keto chocolate cake warm, or store covered on your counter or in the refrigerator (icing will harden).

KETO TEXAS SHEET CAKE WITH CHOCOLATE AVOCADO FROSTING

calories	Protein	Fats	Fiber	Carbohydrates
208	4g	18g	4g	8g

Prep time (start to end): 45 minutes

Servings: 12

INGREDIENTS

TEXAS SHEET CAKE

- 1/2 cup coconut oil, melted
- 1/2 cup cold-brewed coffee (recipe here)
- 3 tablespoons cacao powder
- 1/2 teaspoon cinnamon
- 1 cup almond flour
- 1/2 cup coconut flour
- 1 teaspoon baking soda
- 1/4 cup liquid monk fruit extract

- 1 teaspoon vanilla extract
- "Buttermilk" (1/2 cup almond milk + 1 1/2 tablespoons apple cider vinegar)
- 2 eggs

CHOCOLATE AVOCADO FROSTING

- 1/2 large avocado (about 3 tablespoons)
- 2 tablespoons cacao powder
- 1 tablespoon coconut oil
- 1/4 cup unsweetened lite coconut milk (or dilute 1/8 cup full-fat coconut milk with 1/8 cup water)
- 2 teaspoons liquid monk fruit extract

HOW TO MAKE

1. Preheat the oven to 400 degrees.
2. In a small mixing bowl, combine coconut oil, cold brew, cacao powder, and cinnamon.
3. In a large mixing bowl, combine the almond flour, coconut flour, baking soda, and monk fruit extract.
4. In the small mixing bowl, whisk together the "buttermilk" (almond milk + apple cider vinegar), eggs, and vanilla extract, then add to the mixture in the large mixing bowl.
5. Mix everything until completely combined. You may use an electric mixer, but this works just as well mixing by hand.

6.   Add the batter to a 9×13 baking dish and bake for 20 minutes.

7.   Once finished, remove from the oven and allow to cool while you make the frosting.

8.   Combine all frosting ingredients and mix with a mixer, blender/food processor, or by hand until completely smooth.

9.   Once the cake is completely cooled, spread the frosting, then cut into slices.

LOW-CARB BLUEBERRY CUPCAKES

Calories	Protein	Fats	Fiber	Carbohydrates
138	4.4g	11.4g	1.8g	4.62g

Prep time (start to end): 36 minutes

Servings: 12

INGREDIENTS

- 110 g butter melted
- 4 tbsp. granulated sweetener of choice or more to taste
- 50 g coconut flour
- 1 tsp baking powder
- 1 tsp vanilla
- 2 tbsp. lemon juice
- 2 tbsp. lemon zest
- 8 eggs - medium
- 120 g fresh blueberries

HOW TO MAKE

1. Mix the melted butter, sweetener, coconut flour, baking powder, vanilla, lemon juice, and zest.
2. Add the eggs, one at a time, mixing between each addition.
3. Taste the cupcake batter to ensure you have used enough sweetener and flavors to mask the subtle taste of coconut from the coconut flour.
4. Divide the mixture between 12 cupcake cases.
5. Press in a few fresh blueberries in the batter of each cupcake.
6. Bake at 180C/350F for 15 minutes, or until golden on the outside, and cooked in the center. Ovens will vary so test as the cupcakes are baking.
7. Cover with sugar-free ream cheese frosting. Vanilla or lemon flavor is perfect. Garnish with fresh blueberries and lemon zest.

LOW CARB KETO CUPCAKES

calories	Protein	Fats	Fiber	Carbohydrates
66	1g	5g	2g	7g

Prep time (start to end): 32 minutes

Servings: 1

INGREDIENTS

- 1/3 cup coconut flour
- 1/2 cup unsweetened cocoa powder
- 1/4 cup powdered erythritol (another low carb sweetener of your choice will work)
- 1 teaspoon baking powder
- 1/2 teaspoon baking soda
- 1/4 teaspoon salt
- 4 whole eggs
- 1 teaspoon vanilla extract
- 8 drops stevia extract optional for extra sweetness
- 4 Tablespoons extra light olive oil
- 1/2 cup unsweetened almond milk (or another dairy-free alternative)

HOW TO MAKE

1. Preheat oven to 350 degrees F. Prepare a muffin tin by greasing or baking with cupcake liners.

2. In a medium bowl whisk together coconut flour, cocoa powder, erythritol, baking powder, baking soda, and salt.

3. Make a well in the center of dry mixture. Add eggs, vanilla extract, stevia (if adding), olive oil and almond milk. Mix until ingredients are well combined. Allow to sit for 5-8 minutes.

4. If mixture becomes thicker in consistency than you'd like feel free to add 2 Tablespoons of water to the batter until it reaches your desired consistency.

5. Spoon 2 Tablespoons of batter into each tin. Bake 20-22 minutes, or until a toothpick comes out clean.

6. Frost with your favorite low carb frosting and enjoy!

NO-BAKE COCONUT COOKIES

calories	Protein	Fats	Fiber	Carbohydrates
328.9	2.1g	29.6g	4.9g	4.1g

Prep time (start to end): 10 minutes

Servings: 8

INGREDIENTS

- 3 cups unsweetened shredded coconut
- 3/8 cup coconut oil
- 1/2 cup xylitol (or whatever sweetener you like--see Recipe Notes)
- 2 tsp vanilla
- 3/8 tsp salt (adjust amount as desired)

OPTIONAL TOPPINGS

- Homemade Chocolate / Carob Chips (melted for drizzle)
- coconut shreds
- finely-chopped nuts

HOW TO MAKE

1. Put all ingredients in a food processor or blender.

2. Combine until the mixture is blended and sticks together. (Note: if you are using a high-powered blender like a Vitamix, do not turn your machine on high. You will likely end up with Coconut Butter. While it will be delicious, it won't be these no-bake cookies

3. Remove the mixture from the blender/food processor and form into the desired shape. I like the cute little shapes I was able to make with this little cookie scoop. I had a little trouble with the "balls" falling apart but just gently press them back into the desired shape.

4. Decorate with shredded coconut, cocoa or carob powder, crushed nuts, or melted chocolate (I used my Homemade Chocolate OR Carob Chips, piped from a plastic baggie with a tiny hole cut in the corner) as desired. Or leave them plain. They are great just as is (but I do think a little coconut sprinkled on top adds a nice touch.

5. Leave to firm up on a plate. They will firm up at room temperature.

6. You don't need to store these in the fridge but I think they taste a tad bit better cold.

WHITE CHOCOLATE AND RASPBERRY KETO CAKE

calories	Protein	Fats	Fiber	Carbohydrates
323	4g	31.5g	3.2g	6.6g

Prep time (start to end): 80 minutes

Servings: 8

INGREDIENTS

CAKE:

- 5 ounces cacao butter, melted
- 2 ounces grass-fed ghee
- 1/2 cup coconut cream
- 1 cup green banana flour
- 3 teaspoons pure vanilla extract or 2 teaspoons vanilla powder
- 4 eggs
- 1/2 cup your choice granulated sweetener, such as Lakanto MonkFruit
- 1 teaspoon baking powder
- 2 teaspoons apple cider vinegar
- 2 cup raspberries

WHITE CHOCOLATE SAUCE:

- 3 1/2 ounces' cacao butter
- 1/2 cup coconut cream
- 2 teaspoons pure vanilla extract
- Pinch of salt

HOW TO MAKE

CAKE:

1. Preheat oven to 280 degrees.
2. Combine all dry ingredients until thoroughly mixed through.
3. Leaving the raspberries aside, add all of the remaining ingredients and mix until well combined.
4. Line a small, 8-inch cake or loaf tin with baking paper, and pour in the cake mix.
5. Scatter the raspberries (reserving some for garnishing) over the top of the cake mix. As the cake bakes, they will sink towards the bottom of the cake.
6. Place in your oven and bake for 1 hour, or until firm.
7. While it bakes, prepare the sauce.

SAUCE:

1. Combine all ingredients in a saucepan on low heat.

2. Use a fork to mix all ingredients well to ensure the cacao butter combines with the cream.

3. Remove from the heat and set aside to cool to room temperature. If it's too cool, it will harden, and if it is too warm, it will be slightly runny.

4. Drizzle on each piece of cake when serving, or drizzle over the top of the entire cake if this is what you prefer.

5. Scatter the cake with extra raspberries, and serve.

GLUTEN-FREE CHOCOLATE COCONUT CUPCAKES

Calories	Protein	Fats	Fiber	Carbohydrates
183	4g	21.6g	3.8g	5.7g

Prep time (start to end): 50 minutes

Servings: 15

INGREDIENTS

CUPCAKES:

- 1 cup coconut flour, sifted
- 250g grass-fed butter or ghee
- Pinch of salt
- 7 large eggs or 8 small-medium sized eggs
- 1/2 cup cacao butter
- 1/2 cup cocoa powder
- 1/2 tsp. baking soda
- 1/2 tsp. paleo baking powder
- 1 tsp. apple cider vinegar
- 2 tsp. vanilla powder
- 2 tsp. cinnamon

- 1 cup of xylitol or sweetener of choice

ICING:

- 1/4 cup cacao butter
- 1/4 cocoa powder
- Pinch of salt
- 2-3 tbsp. Brain Octane Oil
- 1/3 cup coconut cream
- Xylitol or sweetener of choice

GARNISH:

- Fresh berries

HOW TO MAKE

1. Preheat the oven to 350°F (170°C). Line two trays of muffin tins with paper cups.
2. Add the cacao powder and butter to a small saucepan and heat over low to medium heat until completely melted and incorporated.
3. Add all ingredients to a food processor and blend until smooth and creamy.
4. Taste the mixture and adjust if needed; adding a touch of extra sweetener of your choice, cinnamon, vanilla, or a little more salt to enhance the chocolate flavor.
5. Spoon the mixture into the pre-prepared muffin trays evenly.

6. Place in the oven and bake for roughly 20 minutes.

7. While the cupcakes bake, add all the icing ingredients to a small saucepan and melt on a low to medium heat until completely combined.

8. Taste the icing mixture and adjust the sweetness if needed. Pour into a bowl, then place in the fridge to set.

9. When the muffins are golden brown and cooked through, remove them from the oven and let them cool.

10. Remove the chilled icing from the fridge. As an optional step, scoop the icing out and re-blend to create a lighter and fluffier icing. Spread over the tops of the cooled muffins and garnish with berries.

11. Store in the fridge.

CHOCOLATE MINT CUPCAKES WITH CHOCOLATE PEPPERMINT SWIRL FROSTING

calories	Protein	Fats	Fiber	Carbohydrates
238.5	2.0g	7.6g	1.2g	41.9g

Prep time (start to end): 30 minutes

Servings: 8

INGREDIENTS

CHOCOLATE CUPCAKES (DAIRY-FREE)

- 3/4 cup coconut butter warm
- 2/3 cup sweetener of choice Monkfruit Sweetener (see link below in Recipe Notes or preferred low-carb sweetener) works for Keto, honey for GAPS/Paleo, coconut sugar/maple syrup also work for Paleo

- 1/2 cup coconut oil melted and warm, or other liquid fat: melted warm butter/ghee, melted warm lard, avocado oil
- 1/2 cup cocoa powder fair trade, see Recipe Notes for link to good cocoa
- 2 eggs room temperature (not cold); you can do this by placing cold eggs in a glass with hot tap water for 30 minutes
- 1/4 cup coconut flour
- 1/4 cup full-fat coconut milk warm (not cold), or full-fat dairy raw milk, if tolerated
- 1 teaspoon gelatin see link in Recipe Notes
- 1 teaspoon peppermint oil optional (You can make the cupcakes plain chocolate if you wish.)
- 1/2 teaspoon baking soda, sifted
- 1/4 teaspoon sea salt

CHOCOLATE MINT SWIRL FROSTING (CONTAINS DAIRY)

- 1 cup butter room temperature (2 sticks)
- 4 ounces' cream cheese or chevre (pour off any liquid), room temperature; okay to replace with butter for GAPS
- 1/3 cup sweetener confectioners Swerve for Keto (or stevia, to taste), honey for GAPS, honey or maple syrup for Primal
- 3 Tablespoons cocoa powder fair trade, see Recipe Notes
- 1 teaspoon peppermint oil see Recipe Notes; brands vary in intensity, so see Recipe Notes for brand or taste for quantity if using a different brand
- 1/2 teaspoon spirulina

HOW TO MAKE

CUPCAKES

1. Preheat oven to 325 degrees Fahrenheit. Place liners in muffin pans. Set aside.
2. Place warm and room temperature (no cold) liquid ingredients in a large bowl and mix: coconut butter, (sweetener if doing GAPS or maple syrup variation), melted coconut oil, eggs, full-fat milk, and optional peppermint oil.
3. In a medium-size bowl, stir together dry ingredients: sweetener (if doing Keto or coconut sugar version), cocoa powder, coconut flour, gelatin, baking soda, and sea salt.
4. Add dry ingredients to wet ingredients. Stir to combine; do not over-mix. Scoop about 2 ounces' batter into each muffin slot.
5. Bake in preheated oven 25 minutes. Test for doneness with a toothpick; look for moist crumbs adhering. Remove from the oven. Cool.

CHOCOLATE MINT SWIRL FROSTING

1. Place in large mixing bowl: room temperature butter and room temperature cream cheese. Use a mixer on high speed to beat together well, until the texture is lightened, about 30 seconds.
2. Add sweetener of choice and continue to beat until well incorporated.

3. Add peppermint oil and spirulina. Mix again until fully incorporated. Scoop half or slightly less than half the frosting into half (taking care to keep it to one side) of a pastry bag (or fully into one pastry bag if you wish to nest 2 full pastry bags inside a third pastry bag to create the swirl).

4. Add cocoa to the frosting bowl. Beat to mix, until fully incorporated. Fill the second-half side of pastry bag with chocolate frosting; (or fill the second pastry bag with chocolate frosting).

5. Pipe frosting onto cooled cupcakes. Serve!

KETO FLOURLESS

CHOCOLATE CAKE

calories	Protein	Fats	Fiber	Carbohydrates
295	6g	26g	5g	8g

Prep time (start to end): 45 minutes

Servings: 12

INGREDIENTS

- 1/3 cup water
- 1/4 teaspoon salt
- 1/2 cup low carb sugar substitute
- 12 ounces unsweetened baking chocolate
- 2/3 cup butter or ghee, cut into tablespoon-size pieces
- 4 large eggs
- boiling water

HOW TO MAKE

1. Line bottom of 9-inch springform pan with parchment paper.
2. In a small pot, heat water, salt, and Swerve over medium heat until salt and sweetener are dissolved.

3. Melt baking chocolate in a double boiler or microwave.

4. Mix melted chocolate and butter in large bowl with electric mixer.

5. Beat in the hot water mixture.

6. Add in egg, one at a time, beating well after adding each.

7. Pour mix into prepared springform pan. Wrap outside well with foil.

8. Place springform pan in larger cake pan and add boiling water to the outside pan about 1 inch deep.

9. Bake cake in a water bath for 45 minutes at 350°F. Remove and cool slightly on wire rack.

10. Chill cake overnight in the refrigerator. Then remove the side of the springform pan.

KETO PROTEIN CHOCOLATE CHIP COOKIES

calories	Protein	Fats	Fiber	Carbohydrates
128	4.5g	11g	2.4g	1.6g

Prep time (start to end): 45 minutes

Servings: 16

INGREDIENTS

- 2 cups blanched organic almond or hazelnut meal
- 3 tbsp. grass-fed Bulletproof Ghee or butter
- 3 tbsp. Bulletproof Collagen Protein
- Stevia or birch tree-sourced xylitol to taste
- 2 tsp. vanilla
- 1 pastured egg
- 1/2 tsp. paleo baking powder
- 1 tsp. apple cider vinegar
- A pinch of salt
- 1/3 cup high quality, sugar-free chocolate, chopped

HOW TO MAKE

1. Preheat the oven to 170°C/340°F. Grease and line two baking trays with parchment paper.
2. Add the almond meal, collagen protein, salt, and baking powder into a bowl.
3. Pour the apple cider vinegar directly on top of the baking powder and allow it to react (it will go fizzy).
4. Add the remaining ingredients to the bowl and stir to combine evenly.
5. Taste the dough and adjust the sweetness if needed.
6. Begin rolling the mixture into balls and place them onto the lined baking tray.
7. Press the balls as flat as you like, they won't rise much, so if you like them softer and chewier keep them quite full. However, if you like a crunchier cookie, press them quite flat using your hands to shape them.
8. Place the cookies in the oven and bake for 15 minutes, or until golden brown.
9. Remove from the oven when they're ready and place the cookies on a wire cooling rack.
10. Store in an airtight container when completely cooled.

COCONUT BLONDIES

calories	Protein	Fats	Fiber	Carbohydrates
189	4g	17g	4g	2g

Prep time (start to end): 80 minutes

Servings: 8

INGREDIENTS

- 1/2 cup (113g) Butter, unsalted softened
- 1/2 cup (105g) Erythritol or sugar substitute
- 4 Eggs
- 1/2 cup (56g) Coconut Flour
- 1/4 cup (56g) Coconut Milk
- 1/2 cup (30g) Desiccated Coconut unsweetened
- 1 tablespoon vanilla extract
- 1/4 teaspoon baking powder
- 1/4 teaspoon salt

HOW TO MAKE

1. Preheat the oven to 180C/350F degrees

2. Grease and line an 8-inch baking pan with parchment paper.

3. In a bowl, cream the butter and erythritol together until smooth.

4. Add the eggs, mixing into the batter, one a time.

5. Then add the vanilla extract and coconut milk and beat until smooth.

6. Next, add the coconut flour, desiccated coconut, baking powder, and salt. Stir until smooth.

7. If the mixture is a bit too thick, add more coconut milk (coconut flour can vary between brands).

8. Spoon into the baking tin and bake for 25-30 minutes until firm and golden.

9. Allow to cool in the tin for at least 30 minutes.

10. Cut into squares and enjoy!

LOW CARB COCONUT MACADAMIA BARS

Calories	Protein	Fats	Fiber	Carbohydrates
199	3.1g	19.3g	2.1g	4.3g

Prep time (start to end): 70 minutes

Servings: 16

INGREDIENTS

CRUST:

- 1 1/4 cups almond flour
- 1/3 cup Swerve Sweetener
- 1/4 tsp salt
- 1/4 cup butter chilled and cut into small pieces

FILLING:

- 1/4 cup butter
- 1/2 cup Swerve Sweetener
- 1/2 cup coconut cream (thick part from the top of a can of coconut milk)
- 1 1/3 cup flaked coconut

- 3/4 cup macadamia nuts chopped
- 1 egg yolk
- 1/2 tsp vanilla extract

HOW TO MAKE

CRUST:

1. Preheat the oven to 350F. Combine almond flour, sweetener, and salt in a food processor. Pulse to combine. Sprinkle the butter over and continue to pulse until the mixture resembles fine crumbs.
2. Press the mixture evenly into the bottom of an 8-inch square pan and bake 15 minutes or until light golden brown. Set aside and let cool while preparing the filling.

FILLING:

1. In a small saucepan over medium heat, melt the butter. Whisk in the sweetener and the coconut cream until smooth.
2. Stir in the coconut, macadamia nuts, egg yolk, and vanilla extract until well combined. Pour the filling over the crust.
3. Bake 35 to 40 minutes, until the edges, are golden brown. Remove from the oven and let cool completely before cutting into bars. The center will not seem set but it will firm up as it cools.

PALEO KETO SHORTBREAD COOKIES

Calories	Protein	Fats	Fiber	Carbohydrates
375	14g	29.5g	7.7g	17.6g

Prep time (start to end): 80 minutes

Servings: 24

INGREDIENTS

SHORTBREAD INGREDIENTS:

- 1 1/3 cup (145g) almond flour
- 1/4 teaspoon fine sea salt
- 1/3 cup plus 1 teaspoon (80g) grass-fed butter or ghee
- 4 tablespoons (40g) erythritol monk fruit blend, such as Lakanto
- 1/2 teaspoon vanilla extract
- 1 tablespoon (8g) coconut flour
- 1 tablespoon (8g) collagen peptides
- 1 vanilla shortbread collagen protein bar, crumbled

CHOCOLATE GLAZE INGREDIENTS (OPTIONAL):

- 4.75 ounces (134g) quality dark chocolate (at least 85% cacao), chopped
- 3 tablespoons avocado oil
- 2 scant tablespoons cacao nibs

HOW TO MAKE

1. In a food processor, mix all shortbread ingredients except for the collagen bar until combined.
2. Remove and spread the dough carefully with a rolling pin until it is about 3.5mm thick.
3. Cut out cookies with curly round cutter and freeze for 30 minutes.
4. Preheat oven to 350 degrees and prepare a perforated baking tray with parchment or a silicone liner.
5. Remove cookies from the freezer, place on the baking sheet, and bake for about 8 minutes, or until golden. Baking time will vary depending on your oven, baking tray, and cookie thickness.
6. Allow shortbread to cool completely before adding glaze.
7. While cookies cool, prepare the glaze: Using a double boiler on the stovetop, gently melt chocolate and oil together until well combined. Mix in cacao nibs.
8. Drizzle cooled cookies with the chocolate glaze and sprinkle with collagen bar crumbs.

KETO LEMON BARS

Calories	Protein	Fats	Fiber	Carbohydrates
272	8g	26g	6g	4g

Prep time (start to end): 60 minutes

Servings: 8

INGREDIENTS

- 1/2 cup butter, melted
- 1 3/4 cups almond flour, divided
- 1 cup powdered erythritol, divided
- 3 medium lemons
- 3 large eggs

HOW TO MAKE

1. Mix butter, 1 cup almond flour, 1/4 cup erythritol, and a pinch of salt. Press evenly into an 8×8″ parchment paper-lined baking dish. Bake for 20 minutes at 350° F. Then, let cool for 10 minutes.

2. Into a bowl, zest one of the lemons, then juice all 3 lemons, add the eggs, 3/4 cup erythritol, 3/4 cup almond flour & pinch of salt. Combine to make filling.

3. Pour the filling onto the crust & bake for 25 minutes.

4. Serve with lemon slices and a sprinkle of erythritol.

54

GLUTEN-FREE & KETO

OREO COOKIES

Calories	Protein	Fats	Fiber	Carbohydrates
86	1g	8g	1g	2g

Prep time (start to end): 35 minutes

Servings: 24

INGREDIENTS

COOKIES

- 144g almond flour
- 37g cocoa powder
- 13g black cocoa powder or simply more regular cocoa
- 3/4 teaspoon kosher salt
- 1/2 teaspoon xanthan gum
- 1/2 teaspoon baking soda
- 1/4 teaspoon espresso powder or instant coffee (optional)
- 80g unsalted grass-fed butter at room temperature
- 128g erythritol
- 1 egg

VANILLA CREAM FILLING

- 56g unsalted grass-fed butter
- 14g coconut oil *
- 1 1/2 teaspoon vanilla extract
- pinch kosher salt
- 63-125g powdered erythritol or powdered sweetener, to taste (we use)

HOW TO MAKE

1. Add almond flour, cocoa powder, xanthan gum, salt, baking soda and espresso powder (optional) to a medium bowl. Whisk until thoroughly combined and set aside.
2. Begin to cream butter in a large bowl with an electric mixer, 1-2 minutes. Add in sweetener and continue to beat until thoroughly mixed and much of the sweetener has dissolved (3-5 minutes).
3. Add in egg, mixing until just incorporated. The mixture will appear slightly 'broken' (i.e. not thoroughly smooth).
4. With your mixer on low, add in half of your flour mixture-mixing until just incorporated. Mix in the rest.
5. Wrap cookie dough with cling film (saran wrap) and refrigerate for 1 hour (or overnight).
6. Preheat oven to 350°F/180°C and line a baking tray with parchment paper.

7. Roll out the dough between two pieces of parchment paper until nice and thin. Cutout the rounds (Oreos are roughly 1 3/4 inches in diameter).

8. Transfer cutout cookies onto prepared baking tray and place in the freezer for 15 minutes before baking.

9. Bake for 8-12 minutes. Since the cookies are dark already and you can't guide yourself by color, we suggest doing a trial with one cookie if possible. When ready, the cookies will have puffed somewhat and smell amazing (this is our best cue here), but you'll want to push the baking time to get them nice and crisp. So just keep an eye out for them.

10. Allow to cool for ten minutes before transferring to a cooling rack. Allow to cool completely, as they'll continue to crunch up (because of the sugar alcohol, this may take a few hours!).

11. To make the vanilla cream filling, cream butter and coconut oil (or more butter) in a medium bowl with an electric mixer. Add in vanilla extract and a pinch of salt, and mix until fully incorporated. Add powdered sweetener to taste and mix until fully incorporated and light and fluffy in texture.

12. Spread or pipe vanilla cream onto a cookie and sandwich between a second one. Refrigerate until set.

13. The cookies themselves keep well, stored in an airtight container at room temperature, for 5 days to a week. Once you add the filling, keep them refrigerated in an airtight container for up to 3 days. The shaped dough can be frozen for up to 3

months, and they can be baked straight from the freezer (adding 2-3 minutes more to the baking time)

KETO CHOCOLATE ICE CREAM

Calories	Protein	Fats	Fiber	Carbohydrates
177	2.7g	14g	1g	3.7g

Prep time (start to end): 25 minutes

Servings: 1

INGREDIENTS

- 4 pasture-raised eggs
- 4 or 5 pasture-raised egg yolks (in addition to the whole eggs)
- 1 teaspoon lemon juice or apple cider vinegar
- 100 grams (7 tablespoons) grass-fed butter or ghee, melted
- 50 grams (3.5 tablespoons) cacao butter, melted
- 60 grams (6 tablespoons + 1 scant teaspoon) XCT oil
- 50 grams (3 tablespoons + 2 teaspoons) coconut oil, melted
- 50 grams (3.5 tablespoons, or more to taste) granulated sweetener of choice
- 50 ml (just under 1/4 cup) filtered water or ice
- 1/4 – 1/3 cup cocoa powder
- 2 teaspoons vanilla powder
- 1 or 2 teaspoons cinnamon (optional)

HOW TO MAKE

1. Add all the ingredients (starting with 30 grams of your chosen sweetener) into a high-powered blender and blitz together for 1-2 minutes.
2. Taste the mixture and adjust the sweetness by adding a little more if needed.
3. Pour mixture into an ice cream maker and churn for 15-20 minutes.
4. Serve and enjoy this incredibly nourishing and delicious ice cream.

KETO PUMPKIN DONUTS

Calories	Protein	Fats	Fiber	Carbohydrates
110	3g	10g	1g	3g

Prep time (start to end): 25 minutes

Servings: 12

INGREDIENTS

- 2 large eggs room temperature
- 1/4 cup unsweetened almond milk
- 2 tablespoons pure pumpkin puree NOT pumpkin pie filling
- 1 teaspoon vanilla extract
- 2 tablespoons melted ghee OR butter if not paleo
- 1/4 cup granulated monk fruit sweetener, can also use granulated sweetener of choice
- 1 cup super-fine blanched almond flour
- 1/2 tablespoon coconut flour
- 1/4 teaspoon xanthan gum
- 1 teaspoon pumpkin pie spice
- 1/2 teaspoon ground cinnamon
- 1 1/2 teaspoons baking powder
- 1/2 teaspoon baking soda

- 1/8 fine sea salt
- mini donut pan

TOPPING CHOICES:

PUMPKIN SPICE COATING:

- 1/4 cup granulated monk fruit sweetener, can also use granulated erythritol OR SWERVE
- 1 teaspoon pumpkin pie spice
- 1 1/2 tablespoons melted ghee, or butter if not paleo

CHOCOLATE GLAZE:

- 2 ounces Sugar-free chocolate, melted
- 1 teaspoon coconut oil, melted
- 1 teaspoon powdered monk fruit sweetener

HOW TO MAKE

1. In a large bowl, whisk together the eggs, almond milk, pumpkin puree, melted ghee, vanilla, melted ghee & monk fruit sweetener, until smooth and combined.
2. In a separate medium bowl, combine the almond flour, coconut flour, xanthan gum, pumpkin pie spice, cinnamon, baking powder, baking soda, and salt. Slowly add the dry ingredients to the wet ingredients & stir until just combined.
3. Transfer batter evenly into a greased 12 cavity silicone mini donut pan (or drop into mini muffin tins) (filling 3/4 full). (Or

you can also use a 6 cavity silicone donut pan for regular-sized donuts.)

4. Bake in preheated oven 350F for 12-15 minutes (for mini) or (21-24 minutes for regular-sized) until golden brown.
5. Remove pan from the oven and set aside until the donuts are cool enough to handle.

PUMPKIN SPICE COATING:

1. While the donuts are baking, stir together the granulated sweetener and pumpkin pie spice in a small bowl.
2. In a separate small heat-safe bowl, melt ghee (or butter).
3. Take each cooled donut and lightly dunk in melted ghee then roll into the cinnamon/sweetener coating.
4. Repeat with remaining donuts.

CHOCOLATE GLAZE:

1. Add the chopped chocolate and coconut oil to a small heat-safe bowl & melt in microwave. Stir in sweetener until combined.
2. Dip the cooled donuts into the chocolate (double-dip if you want a thicker glaze) and place it in the fridge until the chocolate coating has set.

PALEO KETO

CINNAMON ROLLS

Calories	Protein	Fats	Fiber	Carbohydrates
477	5.6g	45.6g	7.1g	17.1g

Prep time (start to end): 45 minutes

Servings: 12

INGREDIENTS

CINNAMON ROLL INGREDIENTS:

- 2 cups macadamia nuts
- 2 tablespoons ground psyllium husks
- 8 tablespoons coconut flour
- 2 tablespoons grass-fed ghee
- 3 tablespoons monk fruit sweetened erythritol (such as Lakanto), or birch xylitol
- 2 teaspoons vanilla extract
- 4 eggs
- Pinch of salt
- 3 teaspoons Ceylon cinnamon

- 1 1/2 teaspoons paleo baking powder
- 1 tablespoon apple cider vinegar
- 1 batch of Keto Caramel Sauce, chilled

GLAZE INGREDIENTS:

- 4 tablespoons coconut cream
- 2 tablespoons grass-fed ghee, melted
- 2 teaspoons birch xylitol or erythritol

HOW TO MAKE

1. In a food processor or blender, grind macadamia nuts into a fine texture (just before they become too buttery). If they do become buttery, the cinnamon rolls will still bake but will not become very fluffy.
2. Combine all cinnamon roll ingredients except for caramel sauce, then place in the refrigerator to chill for one hour.
3. Preheat your oven to 350 degrees. Line a baking tray with parchment.
4. On a parchment-lined surface, roll out dough with your hands and form a large rectangle.
5. With the back of a spoon, gently spread out the Keto Caramel Sauce over the batter, spreading as close to the edges as you can.
6. Gently roll from the dough into a log and seal the edge.

7. Warm a sharp knife under warm water and slice the log into 10-12 rolls.

8. Place rolls on your lined tray and bake for 25-30 minutes, checking after about 20 minutes for doneness.

9. While cinnamon rolls bake, prepare the glaze. Blend all ingredients in a mixing bowl or blender until combined.

10. Remove keto cinnamon rolls from the oven. Allow to cool before glazing, or serve warm with glaze drizzled on top. Store leftovers covered in the refrigerator.

BAKED GLUTEN FREE

& KETO DONUTS

Calories	Protein	Fats	Fiber	Carbohydrates
140	4g	11g	3g	4g

Prep time (start to end): 40 minutes

Servings: 8

INGREDIENTS

KETO DONUTS

- 64 g almond flour
- 28 g coconut flour
- 1 tablespoon psyllium husk ground
- 1 teaspoon xanthan gum
- 240 ml of water
- 57 g grass-fed butter or coconut oil
- 3 tablespoons erythritol or xylitol*
- 1/4 teaspoon kosher salt
- 3 eggs lightly beaten
- 1 teaspoon vanilla extract

- 1 teaspoon baking powder

CHOCOLATE GLAZE

- 75 g powdered erythritol or powdered sweetener
- 14 g cocoa powder
- 1 tablespoon melted butter or ghee/coconut oil, as needed
- 1 teaspoon vanilla extract
- milk-of-choice as needed

SPECIAL EQUIPMENT

- pastry bag or plastic bag
- donut pan (optional)

HOW TO MAKE

1. Preheat oven to 425°F/220°C. Grease and flour (with coconut flour) a donut pan. Alternatively, line a baking tray with parchment paper and draw circles 3 1/2 inches in diameter.
2. Whisk together in a medium bowl almond flour, coconut flour, psyllium husk, and xanthan gum. Set aside.
3. Heat water, butter, sweetener, and salt in a medium pot (or Dutch oven) until it just begins to simmer. Lower heat to low and add in flour mixture, mixing constantly to incorporate. Continue to cook and stir until the dough pulls away from the pan and forms into a ball, 1-3 minutes.

4. Transfer the dough back to the bowl and allow to cool for 5 minutes. The dough should still be warm, but not hot enough to scramble the eggs. And if you have an instant thermometer, the temperature should be below 125°F/52°C.

5. **Add in one egg at a time**, mixing with an electric mixer at medium/high speed until fully incorporated (if using a stand mixer, use the paddle attachment). Be sure to mix the dough for 2 minutes after adding in the last egg; the final texture should be very elastic. Mix in vanilla extract and baking powder.

6. **Allow the dough to rest** until it comes to room temperature (about 15-20 minutes). I've come to realize this is a very important step to keep your donuts from deflating much post bake; the donuts will rise a bit less but hold their shape better.

7. Spoon dough into a piping bag or plastic bag (no tip needed). Cut out the bottom of the piping bag 2 cm (3/4 inch) wide. Pipe out dough onto donut pan, or prepared parchment paper (staying within the drawn circle). Wet your fingertip and smooth out where the ends meet (for a more even rise).

8. **Bake** for 15 minutes at 425°F/220°C, lower temperature to 350°F/180°C and continue to bake for 17-20 minutes until deep golden. **Do not open your oven door** before the first 20 minutes (or at all if possible!), as choux pastry is notoriously sensitive to drafts. Allow to rest in pan for 10 minutes before removing.

9. Note: if your donuts are browning too much, feel free to tent them with aluminum foil (just be sure it isn't resting directly over them!).

CHOCOLATE GLAZE

1. Sift powdered sweetener and cocoa powder into a bowl. Add in vanilla extract, butter, and milk-of-choice (as needed) until desired consistency is reached. The glaze should be thick, but pourable (I like to use our fingertip here to test for thickness!). Glaze donuts by dunking them onto the glaze (if your tops came out a bit wonky, you can always use the rounder bottoms as your new 'tops'!). Alternatively, feel free to brush with melted butter and sprinkle with cinnamon 'sugar'.
2. These are best enjoyed still warm and freshly glazed, but they keep quite well for a day or two stored in an airtight container at room temperature.
3. NOTE: Please note that keto flours vary tremendously from brand to brand, and of course the size of your eggs- so just try using 2 eggs rather than 3!

CHOCOLATE CINNAMON

KETO DONUTS

Calories	Protein	Fats	Fiber	Carbohydrates
112	3g	6.6g	2.4g	13.6g

Prep time (start to end): 12 minutes

Servings: 5

INGREDIENTS

- 1/2 cup green banana flour, sifted
- 3-4 tablespoons coconut milk
- 2 eggs
- 2-3 tablespoons granulated sweetener, such as non-GMO erythritol or birch xylitol
- 1 teaspoon paleo-friendly baking powder
- 1 teaspoon apple cider vinegar
- Pinch of salt
- 1 tablespoon cacao powder, sifted
- 3 teaspoons Ceylon cinnamon

- 1 teaspoon powdered vanilla bean, or 2 teaspoons vanilla extract
- 1 heaping tablespoon grass-fed ghee or softened butter
- Coconut oil for greasing

ICING INGREDIENTS (OPTIONAL):

- 4 tablespoons melted coconut butter mixed with 1-2 teaspoons coconut oil, OR
- 4 tablespoons coconut cream mixed with 1.5 teaspoons cacao powder, stevia drops to taste, a dash of vanilla extract, and 1/4 avocado (all blended until smooth and creamy)
- Optional garnishes: Shredded coconut, edible rose petals, or cacao nibs

HOW TO MAKE

1. Preheat the oven to 350 degrees. Grease a donut tray with coconut oil.
2. Stir all donut ingredients together until evenly combined.
3. Divide the batter evenly into the donut molds, filling until each one is 3/4 full.
4. Bake for 8 minutes, or until donuts are cooked through.
5. Remove the tray from the oven, then carefully remove each donut and place onto a wire rack.
6. Enjoy warm, or cool thoroughly and top with icing and garnishes of choice (if desired).

7. Serve these keto donuts the same day you make them —
   otherwise, they may dry out.

COLD-BREW MOCHA-COFFEE

PANNA COTTA

Calories	Protein	Fats	Fiber	Carbohydrates
110	2g	7g	2g	5.25g

Prep time (start to end): 15 minutes

Servings: 2

INGREDIENTS

- 1 11-ounce container of Mocha Cold-Brew Bulletproof Coffee
- 1 ¾ tsp grass-fed gelatin
- 1 Tbsp filtered water
- Optional: Sweetener, cinnamon, or vanilla to taste
- Optional Toppings: chopped or shaved bulletproof chocolate, whipped coconut cream or toasted coconut

HOW TO MAKE

1. In a small saucepan, add the gelatin and water and stir to combine. Set this aside for a minute or two to allow it to 'bloom' and thicken.

2. When the gelatin has bloomed, add in ¼ cup of the cold brew mocha and heat on low until the gelatin has completely dissolved.

3. Now add the remaining cold brew and stir to combine. Remove the pan from heat.

4. Pour the mixture into 2 small glass jars, then place them in the fridge to set, which should take 1 to 2 hours.

5. When they're ready, serve and enjoy.

KETO COOKIE ICE CREAM SANDWICHES

Calories	Protein	Fats	Fiber	Carbohydrates
662	25g	51g	4g	6.8g

Prep time (start to end): 45 minutes

Servings: 4

INGREDIENTS

COOKIE INGREDIENTS:

- 2 cups fine, blanched organic almond flour
- 3 tablespoons grass-fed butter or ghee, melted
- 3 tablespoons collagen protein
- Stevia or birch xylitol to taste
- 2 teaspoons vanilla extract
- 1 pastured egg
- 1/2 teaspoon paleo baking powder
- 1 teaspoon apple cider vinegar
- A pinch of salt
- 1/3 cup high quality, sugar-free chocolate, chopped

ICE CREAM INGREDIENTS:

- 4 pasture-raised eggs
- 4 or 5 pasture-raised egg yolks (in addition to the whole eggs)
- 1 teaspoon lemon juice or apple cider vinegar
- 7 tablespoons grass-fed butter or ghee, melted
- 3.5 tablespoons cacao butter, melted
- 6 tablespoons + 1 scant teaspoon XCT Oil
- 3 tablespoons + 2 teaspoons coconut oil, melted
- 3.5 tablespoons granulated sweetener of choice (or more to taste)
- Scant 1/4 cup filtered water or ice
- 1/4 – 1/3 cup cocoa powder
- 2 teaspoons vanilla extract
- Optional: 1 teaspoon cinnamon

HOW TO MAKE

1. Begin with keto cookies. Preheat the oven to 340 degrees. Grease and line two baking trays with parchment paper.
2. Add almond meal, collagen protein, salt, and baking powder into a bowl.
3. Pour the apple cider vinegar directly on top of the baking powder and allow it to react (it will go fizzy).
4. Add remaining ingredients to the bowl and stir to combine evenly.
5. Taste the dough and adjust the sweetness if needed.

6. Roll the mixture into balls and place them onto the lined baking tray.

7. Press the balls as flat as you like. They won't rise much, so press down less if you like them softer and chewier. For a crunchier cookie, press them flatter and use your hands to shape them.

8. Place cookies in the oven and bake for 15 minutes, or until golden brown.

9. Remove from the oven and allow to cool for 5 minutes. Carefully transfer to a wire cooling rack.

10. Prepare ice cream: Starting with sweetener, add all ingredients into a high-powered blender and blitz for 1-2 minutes.

11. Taste the mixture and adjust the sweetness by adding a little more if needed.

12. Pour mixture into an ice cream maker and churn for 15-20 minutes.

13. Scoop ice cream into a container and place in the freezer to set for another 10-15 minutes.

14. Using an ice cream scoop, gently add a spoonful of ice cream onto the base of one of the cooled cookies. Top it with another cookie and gently press the cookies into the ice cream to make sure they stick together. Repeat to make 4 ice cream sandwiches.

CHOCOLATE COOKIE DOUGH KETO ICE CREAM

Calories	Protein	Fats	Fiber	Carbohydrates
715	12.5g	70g	11.5g	2.5g

Prep time (start to end): 20 minutes

Servings: 2

INGREDIENTS

- 2 ripe avocados, roughly diced and frozen
- 13 ounces' coconut cream, frozen into ice cubes
- 1-2 tablespoons water or Brain Octane Oil
- 2-3 tablespoons cocoa powder (or more to taste)
- 2-4 tablespoons erythritol (or more to taste if needed)
- 2 teaspoons vanilla extract
- 1 Chocolate Chip Cookie Dough Collagen Protein Bar, chopped into small squares (you can use other flavors, too)

HOW TO MAKE

1. Remove the frozen coconut cubes and avocados from the freezer and allow them to thaw slightly for 5-10 minutes.

2. Now add all of your ingredients (except chopped collagen bar), starting with 2 tablespoons of erythritol to a blender or food processor and blitz until it becomes smooth and creamy. You may need to scrape down the sides of the bowl and re-blend a few times. If you're struggling to get it to blend into a smooth consistency, add 1 tablespoon of water or Brain Octane Oil very slowly until it forms a smooth ice-cream consistency.

3. Taste the ice cream and adjust the sweetness and cacao if needed.

4. When it's ready, scoop into two bowls, sprinkle the chopped bars on top and enjoy immediately.

STRAWBERRY ICE CREAM

Calories	Protein	Fats	Fiber	Carbohydrates
126.7	2.1g	5.5g	0.6g	18.2g

Prep time (start to end): 140 minutes

Servings: 6

INGREDIENTS

- 2 cans (13.5 ounces') coconut milk

- 16 ounces' frozen strawberries

- 1/2-3/4 cup equivalent sweetener (I used Swerve–sweeten to taste)

- 1/2 cup chopped fresh strawberries (optional)

HOW TO MAKE

1. In a blender combine all the ingredients, except for the fresh strawberries, and blend until smooth. Place the mixture in your ice cream maker and process according to the manufacturer's directions.

2. Add the strawberries right before the ice cream is done to combine.

3. Serve immediately or place the ice cream in the freezer for 1-2 hours to harden

SUGAR-FREE CHOCOLATE BARK WITH BACON AND ALMONDS

Calories	Protein	Fats	Fiber	Carbohydrates
157	4g	12.8g	7.5g	12.7g

Prep time (start to end): 30 minutes

Servings: 8

INGREDIENTS

- 1 9 oz bag Sugar-Free Chocolate Chips
- 1/2 cup Chopped Almonds
- 2 slices bacon cooked and crumbled

HOW TO MAKE

1. In a microwave-safe bowl, microwave the chocolate chips on high for 30 seconds, stir. Microwave for 30 more seconds and stir. Microwave for 15 seconds then stir one last time. You want to make sure you have a few unmelted chocolate chips

leftover when you pull it out of the microwave. Then stir one last time and it should be all melted.

2. add the chopped almonds to the melted chocolate and stir

3. on a parchment-lined baking sheet, pour the chocolate mixture in a thin layer, about 1/2 inch.

4. Sprinkle the crumbled bacon on top of the chocolate and press in with a spatula.

5. Refrigerate for 20 minutes or until the chocolate has completely hardened. Peel the parchment from the chocolate and break into 8 pieces. Store in the refrigerator.

KETO WHITE CHOCOLATE

Calories	Protein	Fats	Fiber	Carbohydrates
169	0g	19g	0g	0.5g

Prep time (start to end): 180 minutes

Servings: 1

INGREDIENTS

- 8oz Cacao butter
- 4-5 tbsp. powdered sugar substitute (I used Swerve)
- Any toppings you want, such as cayenne pepper, almonds, etc.

HOW TO MAKE

1. Heat your cacao butter using a Bain Marie. Once the cacao butter has melted and is a nice yellow color, add in your sugar substitute and whisk until it is all mixed.

2. Pour the mix into molds or a parchment paper-lined baking sheet.

3. Freeze or refrigerate until the chocolate is a nice white color. Approximately 2 hours.

LEMON BLUEBERRY DONUTS

Calories	Protein	Fats	Fiber	Carbohydrates
109	4.22g	10.22g	2.84g	6.32g

Prep time (start to end): 35 minutes

Servings: 8

INGREDIENTS

- 1/2 cup coconut flour
- Sweetener equivalent to 1/2 cup sugar
- 2 tsp baking powder
- 2 tsp lemon zest
- 1/4 tsp salt
- 4 large eggs
- 1/4 cup avocado oil (or melted butter)
- 1/4 cup freshly squeezed lemon juice
- 1/4 cup water
- 1/2 tsp vanilla extract
- 1/2 tsp lemon extract
- 1/2 cup fresh blueberries

HOW TO MAKE

1. Preheat the oven to 325F and grease a donut pan well.
2. In a large bowl, combine the coconut flour, sweetener, baking powder, lemon zest, and salt. Stir in the eggs, oil, lemon juice, water, and extracts until well combined. Gently fold in the blueberries.
3. Fill the donut cavities about 3/4 full with batter and bake 18 to 22 minutes, until firm to the touch.
4. You will get 8 to 10 donuts, depending on the size of your donut pan

CHAYOTE SQUASH MOCK APPLE PIE

Calories	Protein	Fats	Fiber	Carbohydrates
187	2g	16.7g	2.9g	6.6g

Prep time (start to end): 60 minutes

Servings: 16

INGREDIENTS

CRUST

- 1/2 cup butter melted
- 1 1/2 cup almond flour
- 3/4 cup coconut flour
- 4 eggs
- 1 tablespoon whole psyllium husks
- 1/2 teaspoon salt

FILLING

- 5 medium chayote squash
- 3/4 cup low carb sugar substitute

- 1 1/2 teaspoon cinnamon
- 1/4 teaspoon ginger
- 1/8 teaspoon nutmeg
- 1 tablespoon xanthan gum
- 1 tablespoon lemon juice
- 2 teaspoons apple extract optional
- 1/3 cup butter cut in small pieces

TOPPING

- 1 egg

HOW TO MAKE

CRUST

1. Mix crust ingredients to form dough.
2. Separate into two dough balls.
3. Roll each crust ball out into the pie crust.
4. Transfer one crust to a 9-inch pie dish. Smooth out any cracks.
5. Reserve remaining crust for the pie top.

FILLING

1. Peel chayote and cut into slices.
2. Boil sliced chayote until fork tender. Drain. Return to pot.
3. Add cinnamon, ginger, nutmeg, sweetener, xanthan gum, lemon juice, and apple extract to cooked chayote squash.

4. Pour chayote mixture into prepared pie crust. Dot filling with butter.

TOPPING

1. Cover filling with reserved pie crust.
2. Flute edges of the pie crust together and cut slits on the pie top.
3. Brush egg on top crust and sprinkle with additional sweetener, if desired.
4. Bake at 375°F for 30-35 minutes.

CHOCOLATE TART

Calories	Protein	Fats	Fiber	Carbohydrates
314	7.5g	26.3g	3.3g	4.8g

Prep time (start to end): 25 minutes

Servings: 8

INGREDIENTS

- 120 g / 1 1/4 cup almond flour
- 70 g / 3/4 cup unsweetened shredded coconut
- 1 medium egg
- 200 ml 3/4 cup coconut cream
- 50 ml / 1/4 cup coconut oil melted
- 10 drops stevia or more, depending on your sweet tooth
- 2 tbsp. and 1 tsp cacao powder unsweetened
- 1 tsp vanilla essence
- pinch of salt
- small handful of chopped hazelnuts to garnish

HOW TO MAKE

1.   Preheat the oven to 180 ºC.

2.   Mix the shredded coconut, almond flour and the egg with a stick blender or in a food processor until it forms a doughy ball.

3.   Press the dough into a loaf tin lined with baking paper (do not omit the baking paper - it makes life so much easier). It should be ca 2 fingers high on the sides. If you wish, pinch the edge with your fingers to make it look pretty.

4.   Bake the tart base for ca 20 minutes or until lightly browned. Remove from the oven and let cool.

5.   Now make the chocolate ganache. Melt the coconut oil, then stir in the coconut cream, cacao powder, vanilla essence, pinch of salt and the stevia or powdered erythritol. Taste and adjust the sweetener if necessary.

6.   Pour into the cooled tart base and place it in the fridge until fully set (ca 1 1/2 hours).

7.   Before serving, dry-roast some chopped hazelnuts in a pan on medium heat until golden. Sprinkle over the tart and enjoy it.

KETO STRAWBERRY TART

calories	Protein	Fats	Fiber	Carbohydrates
187	5g	16g	2g	7g

Prep time (start to end): 30 minutes

Servings: 10

INGREDIENTS

- 5 egg whites
- 1/3 cup xylitol
- 1.5 cups almond flour the finer the better
- 1 lemon zested
- 1 teaspoon vanilla essence
- 1 teaspoon baking powder
- 100 grams' butter melted and cooled
- 250 grams' strawberries washed and sliced

HOW TO MAKE

1. Preheat the oven to 190C / 374F and grease a non-stick tart tin.

2. Lightly whisk the egg whites until foamy and add the xylitol. Whisk further until combined and soft peaks begin to form (don't worry if they don't, some sweeteners will stop this!).

3. Add all remaining ingredients except the strawberries and fold through until evenly combined.

4. Spoon into your prepared tart tin and top with the sliced strawberries.

5. Bake for 18 - 22 minutes until lightly golden. Serve warm or refrigerated.

FINAL THOUGHT

The ketogenic diet recipes is healthy, effective and backed by science. When done properly, the keto diet has been shown to support weight loss, create more mitochondria in your brain, reduce inflammation, and even combat metabolic syndrome diseases. However, any diet can be good or bad for you, depending on what you put on your plate. If you stick to these diet recipes in this cookbook, you enjoy nourishing keto foods.